Strength Training for Women

Sculpt a Strong & Curvy Body Following Workouts Specifically Designed for Females

Thomas Rohmer

Before You Begin:

Bonus Gift: Free Exercise Demonstration Video

As a thanks for picking up this book, I'd love to give you a free gift exclusive to my readers that'll help you get results even faster!

I created a free video where I personally demonstrate how to perform each and every exercise that's in this book.

With this video guide, you'll be able to ensure that you're doing all of the exercises correctly, which will help you maximize your results in the gym.

Visit the link below to instantly download the video demonstration guide for free!

http://rohmerfitness.com/womenvideoguide

Table of Contents

Introduction:

When you think of strength training or lifting weights, what do you typically think of? You probably think of a male in a gym lifting an insane amount of weight.

Stop. Stop it right now.

This belief that only men can lift weights, while women can only lift water bottles and do cardio needs to stop. Yes, not only *can* women lift weights, but women *should* lift weights. If you want to feel fit and feminine, then there's no other way to go about it.

I get it, it can be intimidating walking into a gym filled with guys and going over to the dumbbell rack to train. Don't worry, I'll share with you how you can overcome that fear. I'll also be sharing with you all of the in's and out's you need to know about resistance training as a female:

- Specific workout routines you can follow
- What to do for nutrition
- Should you still be doing cardio?
- Common lies you've been told about strength training for women (such as the myth of toning, etc.).
- Basics of strength training such as what's a set/rep, progressive overload, eccentric vs. concentric vs. isometric phases of a lift, etc.
- And much more.

It doesn't matter if you're completely new to weight training or have been working out for years, this book will still be of great benefit to you. Let's dive in and get started!

Chapter 1: Why "Just Being Skinny" Doesn't Cut It Anymore

You've probably heard someone say, "Someone better feed that girl a sandwich," or "That girl is so skinny, I bet she never eats to maintain that body." Isn't it so interesting how when someone is overweight, it's rude to talk about his or her weight, but when someone is skinny, go ahead and say what you want!

Talk about that person behind their back, and then praise them for their figure in person. Comment online about how that person needs to eat more, or do whatever else it is that you want. That person is skinny so they can handle it! Here are a couple of things to consider:

- Why do people act like simply being skinny is good enough?
- Then once you get skinny, why do you get made fun of?
- Why is it ok to make fun of someone who's skinny, but not fat?
- Are people who poke at skinny people secretly jealous of them?

Imagine for a second the ideal female body you'd like to have. Who do you usually think of? You probably think of someone who is fit, with firm muscles that aren't too big, and with the right amount of muscle in the right places. You don't think of some rail thin model.

Still, society makes it seem as if being skinny is the ultimate goal, as if it's not possible for you to build any muscle at all. You either have to be skinny or fat. Just starve yourself into being thin! Don't worry about working out or any of that nonsense! Then once you do starve yourself thin, people make fun of you for how frail you look. What a lose-lose!

Luckily, this is where weight training comes into play big time. You see, if you only lose weight by dieting, you'll end up looking flat, skinny, and weak. This isn't the look you want to have. On the other hand, if you implement smart nutrition with a proper resistance training routine, you'll build enough muscle to look fit, and you'll burn fat instead of just losing weight.

This is why "just being skinny" doesn't cut it anymore. Being skinny is settling for way less than what you could have. Think about it. There are some girls out there who are naturally skinny. They can eat whatever they want and not have to worry about gaining a pound. I'm sure that many others envy these girls. However, imagine how much better a skinny girl would look if she added a few pounds of muscle in the right places:

- Her legs would look long and lean.
- Firm arms.
- Sleek shoulders.
- A well-defined back

This looks way better than what most people think happens to a girl when she starts lifting weights:

- Capped shoulders
- Bulging biceps
- Ripped back muscles
- Thick tree trunk legs

This is a common misconception about women and lifting weights, and I believe it's one of the reasons why many women are so hesitant to start lifting weights in the first place. Sadly, with all of these lies being talked about, it makes it even harder and confusing to get in shape. Time to put an end to that right now...

Chapter 2: 5 Lies You've Been Told About Women and Lifting Weights

Early on during my fitness journey, I fell for a lot of the lies and myths that are out there. It's frustrating because you end up wasting a lot of your time on ideas that don't work at all. For example, I (falsely) believed that you had to have a body fat percentage of 6% to have good-looking abs. So what did I do? I went all out. I started a crazy diet that consisted of the following:

- Six small meals a day
- Each meal had to contain less than 250 calories per meal
- Each meal had to contain less than 10% of the total calories from fat.
- I never ate anything unhealthy—ever.
- I only drank water.

And on top of this crazy nutrition plan, I went hard with my training in the gym as well:

- 3 days per week I did an intense circuit-training workout.
- Another 3 days per week I did a vertical jump-training workout.
- I went online and made a list of exercises I could do on my "off day."
- And of course, lots of high-intensity cardio!

Did all of this hard work pay off and get me the ripped six pack abs I had been hoping for? No, not even close. In fact, something happened that almost made me quit working out entirely.

It was another hot summer day in Texas, and I was doing another one of my circuit training workouts in my garage with no air conditioning. I was feeling a little woozy because I was restricting my calories to dangerously low levels, and I nearly blacked out while doing a set of jump squats. Now, I'm not one to quit and give up easily, but I felt so bad that I stopped my workout and called it a day.

I contemplated quitting fitness and working out all together—all because I was told the wrong information! Instead of quitting, I decided that I needed to figure out a different approach to nutrition and training. I needed something that would allow me to get in killer shape, but not be so overwhelming that I would be a slave to fitness.

I wanted the best of both worlds, and you should too! And the approach I discovered will allow you to do that. But before I get into the exact methods, let's bust some common myths that surround women and strength training:

Lie #1: Lifting weights will make you look bulky

Are you afraid of working out because you're afraid of looking like a man? If so it's ok, I understand your concern. There are women out there who have a manly looking physique like I described earlier—thick tree trunk legs, capped shoulders, bulging biceps, ripped back muscles, etc. This is far from the ideal feminine physique.

So, how is it that some women achieve this overly muscular look, while others nail it down perfectly? Well for starters, one of the main differences between men and women is hormones. Women have more of certain hormones and less of other hormones than men do.

One hormone that men have more of is testosterone. In fact men produce on average roughly 8 times the amount of testosterone that women do (1). And testosterone is responsible for many things:

- Hair growth
- Muscle mass
- Bone mass
- Fat metabolism
- Aggressiveness

So basically when it comes to fitness, having more testosterone allows you to build more muscle and burn fat way easier. This is why men get super jacked and can build way more muscle than women can.

How is it then that some women lift weights and end up having a more "manly" physique? Well, some women use synthetic testosterone to help them build more muscle and burn more fat. They might be a competitive bodybuilder, or an athlete trying to win a competition.

However, for the average women looking to get in better shape, taking anabolic steroids is unnecessary. In fact, you can build a better body naturally, without the worry of becoming bulky—better than someone can who's abusing drugs. This should come as a huge relief. Training hard in the gym 3-4 days per week will help you build your best body possible, not make you look like a man.

So don't hold anything back when you're lifting weights in the gym. Put it all on the line, and give it all you've got. That's how you're going to get the best results possible. And as long as you're not taking any anabolic steroids (which you shouldn't be), then you have no reason to worry about building manly, oversized muscles.

Lie #2: You can "tone" your muscles

I'm sure you've been told that it's possible for you to tone your muscles. All you have to do is complete a super high amounts of reps with cute pink-coated dumbbells, and you'll magically turn your arms from flabby to firm.

But what exactly does it mean to tone? Most people think it means that you turn the fat you don't want into muscle, but that's not what happens. Your body can do 4 different things in regards to fitness:

- Build muscle
- Lose muscle
- Gain fat
- Burn fat

What women really mean when they say they want toned arms is that they want to lose the fat and build the muscle necessary to make it look firm. And I'll admit toning is a nice word to sum up that definition, but it technically doesn't exist because your body doesn't turn fat into muscle (2). You can burn fat and build muscle separately from each other, which is how you'd achieve your end goal.

The same goes for your muscle turning into fat. Some people complain that their body has turned against them and turned their muscle into fat. In reality however, they've become sedentary, and your body works by a principle called use it or lose it.

Since your body no longer has any need for the extra muscle mass, you'll atrophy. And then you'll burn less calories because you're no longer exercising, which can lead to fat gain. And no, this isn't "reverse toning." It's just being lazy.

Lie #3: You need a post workout shake to get in shape

Strength training is great regardless of whether you're looking to build muscle or burn fat. And the research does show that having a post workout shake is beneficial for individuals looking to build muscle (3). However, how helpful is a post workout shake when you're goal is fat loss? It's been ingrained in our heads that if you don't take a post workout shake within 45 minutes of working out, then your workout was a complete waste.

Is this true? Who benefits the most from selling this lie? Supplement companies, that's who. They want you to believe that the only way you can get fit is by taking one of their "magical" post workout supplements. However, the research shows that when you workout, your human growth hormone levels (hgh) will increase (4). HGH is responsible for helping your body burn fat, and it also helps you maintain your lean muscle mass (5). Therefore, you don't have to worry about your body eating through your muscle mass after a workout because your HGH will protect it.

And in regards to fat loss, how is it that consuming more calories will allow you to lose more weight? Let's say you burned 300 calories during your workout at the gym. Most people will be feeling pretty good about themselves, and they'll feel that they deserve to eat that 500-calorie post workout shake. If they do this, then they'll be worse off overall because they only burned 300 calories in the gym! Don't be that girl who completely ruins her workout all because she felt like she needed post workout protein!

Lie #4: High reps tone and low reps build muscle

As you learned earlier, there's no such thing as toning. Therefore, the other myth you've been told about higher reps toning and lower reps building muscle is false. The truth is that all rep ranges build muscle; the rep range is what determines the type of muscle you'll build (6).

Lower reps stimulate myofibrillar hypertrophy. This is a true increase in muscle size, and it's a dense and firm type of muscle. The other kind of muscular hypertrophy is sarcoplasmic hypertrophy. This type of hypertrophy is stimulated from higher reps, and it occurs when the sarcoplasm grows faster than the myofibrils.

This type of muscle growth is easier to achieve than myofibrillar hypertrophy, however most people want to achieve myofibrillar hypertrophy because it results in an actual increase in the size of the myofibrils. Needless to say, both types of muscle growth are important, and that's why you should be doing high reps and low reps. And you don't have to get into the nitty gritty of the science to realize that higher reps don't tone—higher reps build muscle just like low reps do.

You might also be wondering, "Don't higher reps burn fat and lower reps build muscle?" This is another common myth. People who want to burn fat will lift using higher reps in the gym, thinking that it'll help them burn more fat. However, remember what I just talked about—all rep ranges build muscle. It's the rep range that determines the kind of muscle you'll build.

Sure, it's possible to indirectly burn fat because working out burns calories, but don't believe that changing up your rep ranges will greatly impact fat loss. Therefore, it's easiest to think of things this way—use your workouts to help you build muscle, and use your diet to help you burn fat. Thinking of things in this manner will help to keep things simple.

Lie #5: You only need cardio to get in fantastic shape

The next time you workout in a commercial gym, I want you to look around and notice something. Where are the fittest girls in the gym working out? You'll notice that the women in the best shape are in the weight section of the gym. What you'll also notice is that most of the females in the gym aren't lifting weights, but instead are they are doing cardio.

This is likely because they've been told the same lies you have about how lifting will make them look bulky, so they decide that cardio is the only way to get fit. Sure, doing cardio will burn calories, but you're much better off lifting weights. This is because doing cardio won't help you build any muscle.

If you only did cardio as your main form of exercise, you'd end up looking flat, skinny, and weak—similar to the person who only diets to lose weight. You *must* lift to build muscle and look as good as you possibly can. There are no shortcuts or ways around this fact.

Chapter 3: Set Goals That Let You Crush It & Find Your Why

How many people know that they need to workout and eat right in order to get in better shape? Everybody knows that! So why is it that so few people are actually able to get into amazing shape? It all comes down to mindset. Having a strong mindset will allow you to execute what you need to do in order to be successful with fitness.

This is why it's important to set goals that'll allow you to keep your focus and vision right where it needs to be. Sadly, when it comes to setting goals, most people either don't do it at all, or they mess it up. Only 3% of people write their goals down (7), and of that 3% how many do you think maximize it's effectiveness?

Unfortunately, most people never even bother to write their goals down. They keep it in their head as a wishy washy idea. Here's the exact step-by-step process you need to take to absolutely crush your goals:

Step #1: The first thing you must do is write your goals down with pen and paper. This will make what you want to achieve real instead of an idea in your head.

Step #2: Next, you need to write your goals down in the present tense as if you are working towards achieving them. Your subconscious mind only recognizes the present, so write your goals down in a language your brain understands.

Step #3: Set a date for when you'll achieve your goals by. This makes it real, and helps to create urgency for achieving your goal. If you don't set a date, then what good does that do you? You'll maybe achieve it one day when you get around to it? Imagine if you were getting married and you didn't set a date for when the wedding would be. How ridiculous!

Step #4: Post your goals where you can easily see them. What good is it to write your goals down, then hide them away where you'll never see them?

Put your goals right where you'll constantly see them, like the background on your desktop, or on a notecard in your wallet. Put them anywhere you can think of that will keep them at the front of your mind.

Step #5: Write your goals down every morning and night. This might seem a little tedious, but it absolutely works. Your mind is always looking for problems to solve. By writing your goals down before you go to bed, your subconscious mind will go to work, trying to figure out how it can achieve that goal. Then you'll write your goals down again first thing in the morning. This way you'll maintain that focus for accomplishing your goal throughout the entire day.

Step #6: Share your goals with other people. This can be scary, but it'll pay off once you do it. Tell your friends. Post it on social media. Don't be afraid to put yourself out there and get what it is that you truly want.

Most people are terrified that they'll look like failures and hypocrites if they tell someone and then don't make it happen. What's worse is to not go for anything in your life and play it safe because you were too fearful of what others would think.

I learned this lesson in high school when we were voting for the class favorite. A girl said that I should vote for her, so I told her I would. Immediately after that, another girl said,

"No Thomas, vote for me!" So right then and there I changed my vote trying to please everyone.

Then one of my classmates interjected and forcefully told me that I should vote for whom I wanted and stop trying to please everyone. And boy was he right. No matter what you try to do in life, there will always be critics. So go ahead and put yourself out there and get what you want!

Step #7: Have multiple goals. Don't be afraid to set more than one goal at a time. You can set as many goals as you like, and if you don't accomplish one by the set date, then pick a new date by which you'll reach it.

Step #8: Set goals other than fitness goals. Yes this is a fitness book, but go ahead and set goals for all areas of your life. Why settle?

Here are a few different examples of how you could write down your fitness goals:

- I have 5 pounds of new muscle on my frame by March 20, 2018.
- I weigh 140 pounds by April 18, 2018.
- I can dumbbell bench press 30-pound dumbbells by April 25, 2018.

Notice how much more powerful these goals sound when you write them in the present tense. Imagine if you said I will weigh 140 pounds by April 18, 2018. Why not go ahead and act like you've already achieved the goal?

Of course, these types of goals are outcome goals, but they're not the only types of goals out there. There are also process goals. Process goals are the things you actually have to do in order to achieve your outcome goal. For example, here are some things you'd need to do in order to achieve a goal of gaining 5 pounds of lean muscle mass:

- Lift weights 3-4 times per week
- Focus on getting stronger with your core exercises
- Eat enough high-quality calories to build muscle

For every 1-outcome goal that you have, you'll want to have at least 3 process goals to go along with it. Think of your outcome and process goals like a mountain. The top of the mountain is the outcome you'd like to achieve—it's where you want to get to. The rest of the mountain is the process—it's what you'll have to do in order to reach the top of the mountain.

Should You Focus More on Your Outcome or Process Goals?

When it comes to your goals, should you focus more on your process or outcome goals? This is a tricky question to answer because you need a balance between both. If you focus your attention solely on the outcome, then you'll lose sight of the process, failing to do what it takes to get the job done. On the other hand, if you only care about the process, you'll question the reason why it is you're doing what you're doing in the first place.

Therefore, focus on the outcome goal when it makes sense, and focus on your process goals when it makes sense. For example, let's say you're running low on motivation to workout one day. It's raining and cold outside, and all you want to do is get bundled up and watch T.V.

During moments like this, it's critical that you remember the outcome goal. This will give you the motivation to workout on days even when you don't feel like it. If you only workout on days when you feel like it, then you'll never get in shape. In this instance, thinking of your process goals will only remind you of all the work you have to do—get dressed, drive to the gym, workout with a bunch of different exercises, drive home, shower, and *then* finally get to watch T.V.

When you think of all of that, it's unlikely you'll get the job done. However, if you instead say to yourself, "No. I'm tired of moseying through life, and I want to look good in a bikini this summer. I must achieve what I know I'm capable of, even on days when I don't feel like it. I want that beach body by summer and nothing is going to stop me!"

Do you notice the big difference there? Doesn't remembering your outcome goals fire you up to complete the process? The reason for this is because of something called the pain/pleasure principle. It says that humans do what they do for 1 of 2 different reasons—fear of pain, or the possibility of pleasure.

Think about it. Have you ever worked at a job you hated for way longer than you should have? I know I did. I was desperate to get a job, any job for crying out loud, so I applied to a bunch of different places. The only place to call me back was a pet store, so I took the job for $8.60 an hour and went on my merry way.

The thing was I didn't enjoy that job very much at all. It wasn't because the pay was bad; it was because I enjoyed health and fitness way more than I did pets. Yet, I stayed at that job for 2 years before I quit. The reason why I didn't quit sooner was because I was afraid of what would happen:

- How would I pay rent?
- Would I be able to find another job?
- Would I be able to afford to eat?
- What would my parents think of me being unemployed?

That's what motivated me to keep going forward with a job I disliked. Not having enough money to pay for basic necessities is quite scary. However, when it comes to working out, there isn't going to be any foreseeable consequence for not working out. You're not going to get kicked out of your apartment, or not be able to afford to eat if you don't workout.

Therefore when it comes to achieving your fitness goals, you must hone in your attention towards the possibility of pleasure. Think of how good it'll feel to be in outstanding shape. Imagine the compliments you'll get from friends and family. This'll be what motivates you to keep moving forward, even on days when you don't think you have it in you.

How to Find Your Why

In addition to writing down your outcome and process goals, another thing you can do to motivate yourself is to find your "why." There's a reason, or multiple reasons, why you want to achieve your fitness goals. Getting to the core of that will fire you up. For each outcome goal that you have, ask yourself why it is that you want to achieve that goal. Try to come up with at least 30 different reasons why you want to achieve your various outcome goals. For example:

Outcome Goal: I have 5 pounds of new muscle on my frame by March 30, 2018.

Why?

- I want to have firm muscles.
- I want to look fit.
- I don't want to look flat and skinny.
- I want to prove to myself that I can do it.
- I want to look good in a bikini this summer.
- I want to set a good example for my family.
- I want to feel energized throughout the day.
- I want to feel confident about myself.
- I want to feel more attractive.
- I want to look good in a slim-fitting dress.
- I'm tired of people making fun of me.

Then once you've come up with all of the ideas that you can think of, ask "why" to your original "why's" 2-3 more times— this will get you to the root of what it is you truly desire. These "why's" that you come up with will be the most powerful and motivating of all. For example:

Original why: I want to feel more attractive.

Why do I want to feel more attractive?

I want to be noticed more by guys.

Why do I want guys to notice me more?

I want to be asked out on more dates.

Why do I want to be asked out on more dates?

So I can be in a relationship.

Therefore, the core reason why you want to feel more attractive is because you want to be in a relationship. Make sure you remember that, as well as your other reasons why, when you're lacking the desire to do what you need to do.

Personally, I write all of my reasons why down on a sheet of paper. I then tape that piece of paper up on my wall right above my computer where I constantly see it. Then when I don't feel like doing something, all I have to do is look at that sheet of paper, and I will instantly be reminded why I need to work harder.

Here are some of my reasons that inspire me to be better with fitness and business:

- I don't want to go back to work at a pet shop.
- Getting made fun of for not being able to bench press 200 pounds.

- I never want to have to take orders from a boss.
- I want to be able to do what I want, when I want, with who I want.
- Getting made fun of for being skinny, saying that I would "blow away with the wind."
- I want to reach my full potential.
- I don't want to stress over finances.
- Receiving 0 offers to play college basketball.
- I didn't give it my all in basketball. I won't do the same with working out or my business.
- Getting a job making $8.60 an hour after I graduated from college.

Typing these reasons out really fires me up, and I know that it'll do the same for you! So write down your goals, your reasons why, and get to it!

Chapter 4: How to Easily Gain Confidence and Avoid Gymidation

Walk into any commercial gym and head over to the weight section, and what will you see? You'll notice that the majority of the lifters in the gym are men, not women. You may see some women lifting weights, but most of the women in the gym will be on some sort of cardio machine.

Some of the women doing cardio are doing so because they think that lifting will make them look bulky. Other women do cardio because they're too afraid to lift weight with a bunch of guys surrounding them.

This is the one of most common fears women have about lifting weights. Once a woman realizes that lifting weights won't make her look bulky, she still might be intimidated about actually doing it because of who she'll be surrounded by. On the surface, this seems like a good reason to avoid lifting weights. However, you're about to learn the root of what's really going on, and what you can do to overcome this fear of working out in front of a bunch of men.

And if you're a woman who's afraid of lifting weights in front of a bunch of muscular men, you're not alone. In fact, there are a lot of men who're scared to lift as well. Some men who are beginners that are just starting out feel intimidated by the jacked and muscular guys. They're afraid of looking stupid, and like they don't know what they're doing in the gym!

I used to be one of those guys. It wasn't until late into my
first semester at college that I started working out at the rec
center. This was a great place to workout at, and it had
everything you could want for a great workout—dumbbells
up to 100 pounds, multiple benches and squat racks, plenty
of different machines, cardio equipment, and basketball
courts.

Sadly, I was too terrified of looking like a lost idiot in the
weight room, so I skipped out. I did workouts with resistance
bands in my cramped dorm room instead. You can imagine
how that went. Eventually I mustered up the courage to go
workout at the rec, and I realized it wasn't nearly as bad as I
thought.

Working out in the weight room won't be that bad for you
either! You might be thinking, "Well that's easy for you to say
Thomas, you're a guy!" Look I get it, but let me ask you
something—throughout the day, do you think more about
your own problems and agendas, or someone else's? Of
course you think about your own problems more!

Sure, if you have a significant other or a family, you think
about their needs as well. For the most part though, you're
wondering about what it is that you need to do. So when you
go to the gym, you are thinking about what exercises you're
going to do, how much weight you're going to lift, how many
sets and reps, etc.

You're not pausing to give thought to what someone else is
doing. Your only concern is the workout you're doing! Could
you imagine going up to someone and saying, "Sir, I really
care about your workout. Please tell me everything you're
doing so I can make sure you're maximizing your results!"

The only person who might say this would be a personal
trainer in the gym, and that might even come across as
offensive. The reason why you don't regard other people's
problems before your own is because of something known as

the egocentric predicament. This states that we struggle to see reality outside of our own perceptions (8). We think about ourselves all of the time, and we think that others are always noticing us too.

In reality though, people are barely paying any attention to us at all because they're too busy paying attention to themselves. Initially when you go to the gym to workout, nobody is paying any attention to you. However, if you're paranoid and all you can do is worry about what others are thinking of you, then soon enough you'll do something embarrassing and give people a reason to pay attention to you.

I understand that simply knowing that nobody cares about what you're doing may not be enough to push you over the edge and go for it. If that's the case for you, then try out some of these different mental techniques and see what works best for you. Ultimately though, it'll come down to you going for it and taking action. And remember, the first time will be the hardest—everything will get easier from there!

Visualization Techniques to Overcome Your Fear

Here are some different visualization techniques you can follow in order to overcome your fear of lifting weights in front of other people at the gym:

Visualization Technique #1: Double Disassociation

Imagine yourself walking into a crowded gym full of guys lifting weights. You might imagine yourself as scared and nervous; this is where disassociation comes into play. You would disassociate yourself from your body by imagining yourself in a movie theater watching yourself in the gym like a scene in a movie.

Picture yourself watching a movie in a theater. The movie you're watching is yourself entering a crowded gym full of guys. This is a single disassociation because you're imagining yourself outside of your body.

However, a single dissociation might not be enough for you to feel completely outside of your body. That's why you'll want to disassociate again and imagine yourself in the control room of the theater where the movie is being played.

Now you're watching yourself, watching yourself playing a scene in the movie. Imagine how confident the character feels in the movie, as if nothing bothers her. She goes about her business smoothly and confidently. Picture how in control she is of her feelings and thoughts.

Once you see the character in the movie acting with total and complete confidence, associate yourself back into the movie theater seat, and then once more again to where YOU ARE in the scene in real life, acting confidently like nothing is bothering you. Make your scene as vivid as possible.

What confident thoughts are going through your head? What do you see? What do you smell? What's your posture like? Imagine all of this and practice it over and over until you become unstoppable!

Visualization Technique #2: Anchoring

Many of our fears and phobias come from a negative anchor. Something bad happened, and now every time you see, hear, smell, or taste that stimulus, you're triggered into remembering or acting out those bad feelings.

For example, let's pretend that you're dancing crazily to a pop song at your parent's house. You get too rambunctious and knock over an expensive vase, breaking it. Now every time you hear that pop song, you get a queasy feeling in your stomach like you're about to get in trouble.

This is known as a negative anchor because you've now anchored that song to a queasy feeling. Fortunately, anchors can be positive as well. To do this, you need to get your mind and body in a confident state. Your shoulders should be back, head up, and stomach in.

A good way to achieve this positive state is to listen to your favorite song that makes you feel good. Once you're in a state where you're feeling strong, confident, and unstoppable, create a repeatable stimulus you can use to associate with that positive vibe. A good example would be to snap your fingers.

So snap your fingers repeatedly while you're in this positive state. Repeat this exercise until you get to the point where all you have to do is snap your fingers in order to feel confident!

Visualization Technique #3: Shifting

What kinds of thoughts go through your head when you're sad, mad, or anxious? Usually negative things like, "I'm no good", "I'm not sure if I can do this", "Why does this always happen to me?" etc. And how is your posture when you're thinking these thoughts?

Your shoulders are slumped, your head is down, and you have a frown on your face. But remember—we're in control of how we think and act. Therefore, we're also in control of how we feel. The first thing you must do is recognize how you're feeling. You must catch yourself in the negative state that you want to change.

When this happens, I want you to imagine a big red stop sign. It should get to a point where every time you think about something negative, the stop sign immediately pops into your head. After this, change your state to a positive one.

Do this by changing your posture—keep your head held high, set your shoulders back, and put a big smile on your face.

After your body is in a positive state, your mind will follow along with it. Have you ever noticed how hard it is to feel unhappy when you have a big smile on your face? It's pretty hard! So next time when you're feeling down or anxious, recognize it, stop it, and then change your physical state!

Visualization Technique #4: The Bathroom Mirror

Don't use your bathroom mirror just to get ready in the morning. It can be used for so much more than that! Use it to help you become unstoppably confident! To practice this technique, stand in front of your bathroom mirror and assume a confident position—head up, shoulders back, stomach in, etc.

Then say positive affirmations to yourself over and over again in the mirror. Your roommates may think you're crazy, but who cares! The trick with this is to say the affirmations with the word "you" instead of "I." This is because the word "you" speaks directly with your subconscious mind, and it's way more powerful than saying "I."

Here are some examples of what you could say to yourself:

- No one can stop you.
- You won't stop until you get what you have to have.
- You become more confident with each step you take.
- You lift weights like it's nothing.
- You're on a mission.

Practice some of these phrases and others you come up with as part of your daily routine to easily feel completely powerful!

Visualization Technique #5: Just a Dot

Whenever something is stressing us out, it consumes us. It controls us if we're not in control. To overcome this, put things in perspective by imagining your entire life on a timeline. Picture the date you were born, and all the time inbetween, down to a predicted date when you'll pass away.

Then imagine this stress or anxiety you're feeling about working out in front of others as a small, insignificant dot on this timeline. In comparison to the rest of your life, it doesn't seem like a big deal does it? And if this isn't enough, then widen your perspective even more.

Picture a different timeline, the timeline of the entire history and future of the universe. Imagine how much smaller your single dot is on THAT timeline. It's absolutely nothing!

And if all else fails, the last tip I have for you is to try working out at a time when the gym isn't crowded, like early in the morning. This might not be the most practical option for you depending on your schedule, but if you can make it work, give it a shot!

Chapter 5: Strength Training Basics You Need to Know

I first started lifting weights when I was 13 years old. I did it as part of the athletics program in my school so I could play sports. I still remember my first day in the weight room—boy was I scared. I was in the 7th grade and I had to lift weights will all of the experienced 8th graders.

The coach briefly explained how to rotate to a different exercise when the timer went off, what a set and rep was, etc. He asked if anyone had any questions, and of course I had a million questions, but I was too afraid to speak up. I had no idea what I was doing, and I felt so lost.

It was a terrible feeling, and I don't want you to go through what I did. I don't want you to go to the gym and feel like a chicken with it's head chopped off. And if you're completely new to resistance training, you're probably unfamiliar with all of the typical gym lingo like I was when I first started. You might hear someone say, "Do 3 sets of 10 reps," and think to yourself, "What in the world does that mean?"

You might even feel embarrassed, but everyone has to start from somewhere. No one was born knowing what an isometric exercise is; they had to learn it at some point. And what better time to learn all of this than right now! Understanding these weight-training basics will allow you to feel confident and crush it every time you go to the gym. So let's dive in and get you familiar with what you need to know!

What's a set, rep, and rest period?

A set is a group of consecutive repetitions. A repetition is one complete motion of an exercise. And the rest period is how long of a break you'll take until you start the next set. For example, let's say you're completing 3 sets of 8 reps and resting 2 minutes in between sets for the barbell squat exercise.

You'll squat down and stand back up, completing the motion of the exercise (one rep). You'll repeat that motion 7 more times for a total of 8 repetitions. That will complete the set, and you will begin your rest period. Once your 2-minute rest period is up, you'll start the next set and perform another 8 repetitions.

That will complete set number 2, and you'll rest another 2 minutes. Once that time period is up, you'll complete the final set of 8 repetitions, and then you'll move onto the next exercise.

Different phases of a lift: eccentric, concentric, and isometric

During any exercise, there are going to be 3 different phases to the lift. There's a concentric, eccentric, and isometric part to every weight lifting exercise that you do. Here's the breakdown of each:

Concentric phase of the lift: This is the part of the lift where the muscle is shortening in length, and it's the part where you're actually lifting the weight. For example, during a bench press, the concentric part of the exercise would consist of you pressing the bar from your chest and fully extending your arms. And during a bicep curl, the concentric phase would occur when you're lifting the dumbbell from resting at your side towards your shoulder.

Eccentric phase of the lift: During this phase of the lift, the muscle is lengthening as you return the weight to its starting position. In the example of the bench press, this would occur when you're lowering the bar back down towards your chest. And with the bicep curl, the eccentric phase would occur when you're lowering the dumbbell down from your shoulder back down to your side.

Believe it or not, you're at your strongest when you're performing the eccentric part of the lift (9). This means that you can lift more weight when you are lowering the weight opposed to when you're lifting it. For example, if you were doing a dumbbell curl, you could control a heavier weight on the way down than you could lift on the way up.

This is why it's critical to control the weight on the way down. Pay attention to the way people lift in the gym. Most people aren't controlling the weight on the way down at all— they simply let it fall. If you mess this up, you'll be missing out on a lot of potential strength and muscle gains.

Isometric phase of the lift: The isometric phase of the lift occurs when the length of the muscle remains unchanged, but there is still tension on the muscle. In the example of the bench press, this would occur at the point when you hold the bar for a second at the top when your arms are fully extended. During a dumbbell curl, this would occur when you're holding the dumbbell at the top position by your shoulder.

What is workout tempo?

The tempo of an exercise refers to how long each phase of the lift will last for. There are a variety of different tempos that you can use depending on what your goals are, but there's one tempo that works great for most fitness goals. A great workout tempo (and the one you'll be using for the workouts in this book) is as follows:

- 1 second (or as fast as you can lift the weight) concentric
- 1 second isometric
- 4-second eccentric

For example, let's say you're performing a squat exercise. You'll squat the weight up as fast as you possibly can, which should only take around 1 second. Then you'll pause at the top for 1 second, which is the isometric phase of the lift. And finally you'll slowly lower the weight (this is the eccentric phase), squatting down over the course of 4 seconds.

Remember, the eccentric phase of the lift is extremely important because that's where the majority of the muscle damage will be occurring. That's why you want to lift using a 4-second eccentric. Most people lift using a 1 second eccentric, which will not give them maximum results, so make sure you're consciously aware of how slow you're lowering the weight.

How Does Your Body Gain Strength?

If you're curling 10-pound dumbbells right now, and you want to curl 20-pound dumbbells, how will you reach your goal? It all comes down to a principle known as progressive overload. This principle states that you must constantly be doing more work, either by increasing the amount of weight you're lifting and the reps you're doing, or decreasing the rest periods in order to gain strength, build muscle, and get results.

Let's say that right now, you're able to do 80 pounds on the lat-pulldown machine for 10 reps. If 3 months later you're still doing 80 pounds for 10 reps, you won't be getting any new results. You must steadily increase the reps and weight you're lifting over time. If you increased your lat-pulldown to 100 pounds over that same 3-month period, you would be making some new muscle gains.

This is why it's important to keep track of your workouts on your phone. You can do this by recording how much weight you're lifting for each exercise, how many reps you're doing, etc. This way you'll know what numbers you need to beat every time you step foot into the gym.

How Does Your Body Build Muscle?

Have you ever gone camping and started a fire? In order to keep the fire going, you must give it more wood. Essentially, you must use the fire, or you'll lose the fire. Your body works off the same principle with muscle. Muscle takes a lot of energy to maintain, so your body will only keep what it thinks is necessary to survive.

When you workout, you breakdown your muscle fibers and send a signal to your body that you need this muscle. Your body will respond by building more muscle to help prepare itself better for the next time you workout. However, if you stop working out, you will stop providing that stimulus to your body, and you'll atrophy (lose muscle).

Of course, working out is only one component to building muscle. The workout will breakdown your muscle, and signal to your body that you need to build muscle. However, it's when you're away from the gym—resting, recovering, and giving your body the nutrients it needs—that your body will build itself back up bigger and stronger.

Think of it like this—pretend you're an architect and you're building a house. In order to build the house the size you want, you'll need 8,000 bricks. If you have an issue with the brick supplier and only end up with 6,000 bricks, you'll have to build a smaller house. It won't be possible to build a bigger house unless you get more bricks.

The same is true with building muscle. Your body needs a certain amount of calories to build muscle (more on this later). If you don't give your body all of the calories it needs, then you'll be leaving muscle on the table so to speak. By combining a solid training plan with a great nutrition strategy, you'll be able to maximize the results you get with building muscle.

Isometric vs. Compound Exercises

One way to group exercises is by classifying them as either isometric or compound exercises. Isometric exercises only work one muscle group. An example of this would be a tricep pushdown. This exercise only works one muscle group—the triceps. Here's a list of common isometric exercises:

- Barbell/Dumbbell Curls
- Tricep Extensions
- Tricep Pushdowns
- Leg Extensions
- Hamstring Curls
- Lateral Raises
- Cable Crossovers

Then there are compound exercises. Compound exercises work multiple muscle groups at one time. An example of a compound exercise would be a leg press. The leg press exercise works on the quads as the primary muscle group, and it also works the hamstrings and glutes as secondary muscle groups. Here's a list of common compound exercises

- Bench Press
- Squat
- Deadlift
- Pull-Ups
- Lat-Pulldowns
- Overheard Press
- Any row variation
- Leg Press

The cool thing about compound exercises is that they work multiple muscle groups at the same time. This means that you'll get more work done in less time. And because you'll have multiple muscle groups working together, you'll also be able to lift more weight than you would with an isolation exercise.

Compound exercises also require more core strength and burn more calories than isolation exercises. At this point, you might be wondering why you should even bother with isolation exercises. Generally, compound exercises are more technical lifts, and it will take longer for you to master your form. This also means you have an increased chance of injury if you're not performing the exercise correctly.

Isolation exercises are much easier to perform, and you can get the form down pretty quickly. They also allow you to target certain muscle groups that usually only get to work as secondary muscle groups. For example, when you do a bench press, the primary muscle group being worked is the chest.

The triceps and shoulders act as secondary muscle groups. So the only way you can make the triceps the primary muscle group being worked is by isolating it, and doing exercises like pushdowns and extensions. For the most part however, compound exercises should be the focus. In the weight training program, you'll notice that the compound exercises are performed first because they're the most important.

You'll typically go heavy with these exercises and do less reps. Isolation exercises still have their place, but they'll be performed after all of the compound movements. You'll usually lift a lighter weight with these exercises and perform a higher number of repetitions.

Different Ranges of Motion

When you're lifting weights, there are 3 different ranges of motion you can lift from: stretch, mid range, and peak contraction. These 3 different ranges of motion determine where most of the tension will be occurring when you lift. In other words, the range of motion will tell you what part of the lift is the hardest. Here's the breakdown of each:

Stretch Exercise: most of the tension with stretch exercises will be occurring at the bottom part of the movement, when you're first starting to lift the weight. An example of this would be an incline dumbbell curl.

Midrange Exercise: most of the tension with a midrange exercise will be occurring during the middle part of the exercise, essentially when you're at the halfway point. An example of a midrange exercise would be a standing dumbbell curl.

Peak Contraction Exercise: most of the tension with a peak contraction exercise will be happening during the top part of the exercise. Peak contraction exercises place your body in a position where the muscle will be fully shortened. An example of a peak contraction exercise is a spider curl.

Note: If this concept confuses you, don't worry about it too much. You don't need to know what the range of motion is for every exercise that you do. It's useful to know if you're interested in working the same muscle from multiple angles.

Breathing While Lifting Weights

Breathing during exercise is not something that a lot of people think about, but it's quite important. This is something you'll get better with over time, so don't worry if you find yourself messing it up in the beginning.

Remember what you learned earlier about the concentric and eccentric parts of a lift. As a refresher, with a squat exercise, when you're squatting down that's the eccentric part of the lift. And when you're standing back up, that's the concentric phase.

The breathing technique you're going to use for each exercise is simple, but it'll take some practice to get the hang of. All you're going to do is exhale during the concentric phase of the lift, and inhale during the eccentric part of the exercise. Using the squat as an example again, you'll breath in while you're squatting down. Then you'll breath out while you're standing back up.

Another example with the bench press would be inhaling while you bring the bar towards your chest. Then you would exhale as you press the bar up and fully extend your arms.

Chapter 6: Setting Up Your Strength Training Routine

Note: Before you get started with this workout routine, be sure to download my free video guide by visiting the link below where I personally demonstrate and show you how to do each exercise found in this book:

http://rohmerfitness.com/womenvideoguide

Now it's time for the fun part. I've gone over the basics you need to know in order to set you up for success. After you have a good workout plan in place, it all comes down to execution. You can workout 3 or 4 days per week. Choose whatever will work best for your schedule. If you're brand new to weightlifting, I recommend starting with 3 days per week and then building your way up to 4.

I'll be providing a workout plan for both beginners and intermediate/advanced lifters as well. So no matter where you're starting from, you'll be able to push yourself and see results!

Beginner's Workout Plan

Follow this beginner's workout plan if you're completely new to strength training, or if you've been lifting weights for less than a year.

This workout will consist of 3 full-body workouts per week. Full-body workouts are great because they allow you to get good at performing key exercises quickly. You'll also be stimulating your muscle groups more often, which will help you to maximize your results as a beginner. Here are a couple of different ways you can set up your workout schedule:

- Monday: Workout
- Tuesday: Rest Day
- Wednesday: Workout
- Thursday: Rest Day
- Friday: Workout
- Saturday: Rest Day
- Sunday: Rest Day

Or:

- Monday: Rest Day
- Tuesday: Workout
- Wednesday: Rest Day
- Thursday: Workout
- Friday: Rest Day
- Saturday: Workout
- Sunday: Rest Day

Here is the actual workout that you'll be doing:

- Leg Press: 3 sets of 10 reps (90 sec rest between sets)
- Incline Dumbbell Press: 3 sets of 8 reps (90 seconds rest between sets)
- Lat-Pulldowns: 3 sets of 8 reps 90 seconds rest between sets
- Standing Dumbbell Press: 3 sets of 8 reps (90 seconds rest between sets)
- Hamstring Curls: 3 sets of 12 reps (60 seconds rest between sets)
- Standing Dumbbell Curls: 3 sets of 10 reps (60 seconds rest between sets)
- Tricep Pushdowns: 3 sets of 10 reps (60 seconds rest between sets)

Intermediate/Advanced Workout Routine

Follow this workout routine if you've been working out for at least 1 year consistently. This workout is going to follow something called a split routine, which means that we'll be splitting up the muscle groups worked between different workouts.

This workout will consist of two different workouts: A and B. You'll alternate between workout A and B each time you go to the gym. During workout A, you'll be working on your leg, back, and bicep muscles. During workout B, you'll be working on your chest, shoulder, and tricep muscles. So the first time you go to the gym to workout, you'll do workout A. The next time you go to the gym, you'll do workout B.

Here's how to setup your workout schedule if you want to workout 3 days per week:

- Monday: Workout A
- Tuesday: Rest Day
- Wednesday: Workout B
- Thursday: Rest Day
- Friday: Workout A
- Saturday: Rest Day
- Sunday: Rest Day
- Following Monday: Workout B

Or:

- Monday: Rest Day
- Tuesday: Workout A
- Wednesday: Rest Day
- Thursday: Workout B
- Friday: Rest Day
- Saturday: Workout A
- Sunday: Rest Day
- Following Tuesday: Workout B

And here's how to setup your gym schedule if you want to workout 4 days per week:

- Monday: Workout A
- Tuesday: Workout B
- Wednesday: Rest Day
- Thursday: Workout A
- Friday: Workout B
- Saturday: Rest Day
- Sunday: Rest Day

Or:

- Monday: Workout A
- Tuesday: Workout B
- Wednesday: Rest Day
- Thursday: Workout A
- Friday: Rest Day
- Saturday: Workout B
- Sunday: Rest Day

Here are the actual workouts:

Workout A: Legs, Back, and Biceps

- Bulgarian Split Squats: 3 sets of 8 reps, per leg (90 seconds rest between sets)
- Reverse Dumbbell Lunges: 3 sets of 8 reps ,per leg (90 seconds rest between sets)
- One Arm Dumbbell Row: 3 sets of 8 reps (90 seconds rest between sets)
- Lat-Pulldown: 3 sets of 10 reps (60 seconds rest between sets)
- Incline Dumbbell Curls 3 sets of 10 reps (60 seconds rest between sets)
- Cross Body Hammer Curls: 3 sets of 10 reps (60 seconds rest between sets)

Workout B: Chest, Shoulders, and Triceps

- Incline Dumbbell Bench Press: 3 sets of 6 reps 2 minutes rest between sets
- Standing Dumbbell Press: 3 sets of 8 reps 90 seconds rest between sets
- Standing Dumbbell Lateral Raises: 3 sets of 12 reps 60 seconds rest between sets
- Bent Lateral Raises: 3 sets of 12 reps 60 seconds rest between sets
- Tricep Kickbacks: 3 sets of 10 reps 60 seconds rest between sets
- Tricep Pushdowns: 3 sets of 10 reps 60 seconds rest between sets

Chapter 7: How Often Should You Change Things Up?

This is one of the most common questions people have about their strength training routines. People wonder how often they should be switching up their workout routine. The simple reality is that you shouldn't be changing up your workout routine as often as most people do.

People get bored easily so they hop from one workout to the next. Maybe they'll try strength training one week, high intensity interval training the next, and circuit training the following week. Jumping ship and dabbling in a little bit of everything is a great way to get no results.

Remember the principle of progressive overload from Chapter 5. In order to build strength and gain muscle (aka get results), you must do more work over time. So for instance, if you can lift 20-pound dumbbells for the incline bench press exercise, and 3 months from now you're still lifting the same weight, you won't be getting any new results.

With that in mind, think of someone who constantly changes up her workout routine. This person doesn't necessarily have to change to some completely different style of working out—she could change up the exercises too often and wreck her results.

Imagine this person is using 15-pound dumbbells for the standing military press exercise. A month later she's doing the same exercise with 25-pound dumbbells. She's making some great progress, but then she gets bored and unnecessarily swaps that exercise out for a different one. How is she supposed to keep getting results with that exercise if she gets rid of it as soon as she gets bored? She doesn't!

This is why so few people in the gym are able to maximize their results. Why not squeeze everything you can out of your current workout before you change it up? That's why you should stick to the same workout plan provided for at least 12 weeks before you consider changing anything.

After that 12-week period you can swap some exercises out if you need to, but keep the same workout structure. For example, if you're doing full body workouts, keep doing full body workouts, just change the exercises.

But remember—if it ain't broke, don't fix it. If you're still making progress with the exercises you're doing, then keep doing them! The only circumstance where you should be switching out exercises is when you hit a plateau. A strength plateau is when you're no longer lifting more weight for a certain exercise. Before I get into the ins and outs of strength plateaus, it's first important to understand how you should be making progress on your lifts:

How Much Weight Should You Lift and When Should You Increase the Weight You're Lifting?

If you're new to weightlifting, you won't know how much weight to use for the given exercises. You'll just have to take your best guess and go from there. For example, let's say you think you can do 100 pounds when the program calls for 10 reps of the leg press exercise.

So you use 100 pounds and do 15 reps easily. This means that the weight is too light and you need to go heavier. The next set you do 115 pounds and only do 8 reps. When this happens, don't worry. It's completely ok.

Just make a note of it in a workout journal (yes you should actually use a workout journal), and then strive to hit 10 reps with 115 pounds the next time. Once you get 10 reps for all 3 sets with 115 pounds, that's when it's time to bump up the weight.

Now with that in mind, let's bring the topic back to strength plateaus. Let's say you build your way up to doing 150 pounds on the leg press. Your goal is to do 10 reps on all 3 sets so you can bump the weight up to 155. On your last workout, you did 150 pounds for 8 reps on the 1st set, 7 on the 2nd, and 6 reps on the 3rd set.

During this workout you want to try and get more than 8 reps on the 1st set, 7 on the 2nd, and 6 on the 3rd with the same 150 pounds. However, let's pretend that you weren't able to beat any of your previous numbers. That's ok, you don't need panic at this point. Try to beat them the next time you do leg press.

If you go 3 workouts in a row where you're unable to improve on your numbers for a given exercise, that's when I would consider swapping it out for a different exercise. Of course you'll want to make sure you switch out leg exercises for leg exercises and chest exercises with different chest exercises. Don't take out a shoulder exercise and replace it with a tricep exercise just because you feel like it.

Here's a list of some interchangeable exercises you can use in your exercise routine. Remember though that you shouldn't change anything for the first 12 weeks. This is especially true if you're a beginner. You shouldn't be running into any strength plateaus during your first 3 months of training. With that being said, here's the list of substitutions; you can simply pick any of the exercises on the list for the given muscle group that you'd like to start doing:

Biceps

- Incline Dumbbell Curls
- Standing Dumbbell Curls
- Cross Body Hammer Curl
- Hammer Curls

Triceps

- Overhead Dumbbell Tricep Extension
- Skull Crushers
- Tricep Rope Pushdown
- Tricep Kickbacks
- Tricep Pushdown

Chest

- Incline Dumbbell Press
- Incline Barbell Press

Back

- Bent Over Rows
- T-Bar Rows
- One Arm DB Rows
- Seated Cable Rows

Legs

- Pistol Squats
- Leg Press (done one leg at a time or normally with both legs)
- Bulgarian Split Squats
- Reverse Lunges

Shoulders

- Standing Dumbbell Press

- Seated Dumbbell Press
- Seated Barbell Press
- Standing Barbell Press
- Cable Lateral Raise
- Seated Dumbbell Lateral Raise
- Standing Dumbbell Lateral Raise
- Reverse Pec Deck Machine
- Bent Lateral Raises

Note: These are just some ideas. This isn't an all-encompassing list.

Chapter 8: Don't Forget About Nutrition!

Although this is a book on strength training, it is important that you do not neglect your nutrition. What you eat will be providing you with the fuel that you'll use during your workouts, and it'll help you recover from your workouts. With that being said, let's go over some basics of nutrition...

What is a Calorie?

You've probably heard of the word calorie before, but you might not be exactly sure what it means. Essentially, a calorie is a measurement for energy. Our body needs energy everyday to complete tasks such as breathing, organ function, digestion, etc. When we eat, we get calories (energy) from the foods we eat.

The total amount of calories we burn off in a given day is referred to as our resting metabolic rate. You can determine your resting metabolic rate by multiplying your bodyweight by 13. Using myself as an example:

Body weight = 200 pounds

200 x 13 = 2,600

This means that 2,600 is my maintenance calories. I won't gain or lose weight if I eat 2,600 calories a day.

If I eat less than 2,600 calories per day, I'll be in a caloric deficit and I'll start to lose weight.

If I eat more than 2,600 calories per day, then I'll be in a caloric surplus and I'll start to gain weight.

This is a crucial topic to understand. If you want to burn fat, then you must eat less calories than your resting metabolic rate. On the other hand, if you want to build muscle, then you need to eat more calories than you're burning off.

If You Want to Burn Fat

If your goal is weight loss, then calculate your resting metabolic rate by multiplying your bodyweight by 13. Then take that number and subtract 500 from it. Here's my example:

Body weight = 200 pounds

200 x 13 = 2,600

2,600 - 500 = 2,100

This means that I need to eat 2,100 calories a day to start losing weight. This will set you up to start losing roughly 1 pound per week since there are 3,500 calories in one pound of fat (10).

Also, you don't need to change up your workouts at all if you're trying to burn fat. The easiest way to control your calories is through your diet. Focus on your workout to make you look lean and fit. Focus on your diet to help you burn off fat. This way when you to lean down, you'll look outstanding instead of flat and weak.

If You Want to Build Muscle

If you want to build muscle, you'll need to eat more calories than you consume. This is because your body needs the extra nutrients to help build your body back bigger and stronger than before. The trick is to not eat too much. Overeating can lead to fat gain, and that's not something we want to happen.

That's why you need to take your resting metabolic rate (13x body weight) and add 250 calories to that number. Here's myself as an example:

Body weight = 200 pounds

200 x 13 = 2,600

2,600 + 250 = 2,850

This will have me building about half a pound of muscle per week. This is the perfect amount to maximize gains, but not gain fat. Most people try to rush the process and end up gaining fat unnecessarily.

The reality is that building muscle is a slow process; don't try to speed it up when you can't. Focus on making progress with your workouts, eat the right foods in the right amounts, and you'll be good to go.

Can I Build Muscle and Burn Fat at the Same Time?

You might be tempted to try and build muscle and burn fat at the same time. It's possible, but only for certain individuals. You'd have to be a complete beginner with some excess fat to lose in order to pull this off. If you're an intermediate to advanced trainee, it's going to be next to impossible to achieve.

The reason for this is that as an advanced lifter, you've already maximized your "newbie gains" that you made when you first started lifting. In addition to that, it's even more critical that you eat in a caloric surplus in order to build

muscle because your body will have less fat stores to feed off
of.

A lot of people end up getting no results at all because they
try to chase two different rabbit holes at the same time.
They'll try to build muscle for a couple of weeks, then they'll
shift gears and try to burn fat.

The best thing you can do for yourself is to pick one goal
(build muscle or burn fat) and stick with it until you reach
your end goal. Once you've built all the muscle or lost all the
weight you wanted to, then move onto the next thing.

For example, let's say you're a complete beginner to strength
training and you have a bit of excess fat you'd like to lose.
You need to only focus on losing the fat. What you'll notice is
that you'll still be able to gain some strength and muscle in
the gym because you'll be taking advantage of what's known
as "newbie gains".

You have so much untapped potential when you start lifting
that your body will grow just because it's so shocked from a
new stimulus. Of course this won't last forever, so enjoy it
while you can. Needless to say, you don't need to worry about
trying to do everything at once as a beginner.

Hone your attention in on the basics. If you're consistently
working out hard in the gym and eating right, you'll get good
results. Conversely, if you're trying to win a figure contest,
then every little detail needs to be on point.

How to Track Your Calories

Let's say you determine that you need to eat 1,700 calories a
day in order to start burning fat. How do you know if you're
actually eating 1,700 calories? Similar to tracking your
workouts in the gym, there will be no way to tell if you're
eating 1,700 calories a day unless you measure it.

This is certainly the most tedious part of nutrition. However, most people never even give the thought to tracking what they eat, and they get sloppy results because of it. The easiest way to track your calories accurately and efficiently is to use a calorie counting app. Download any popular app in the app store for a couple of bucks.

The $3 you'll spend on a calorie counting app will pay for itself many times over. Many of them have barcode scanners where you can simply scan the barcode and it'll automatically add the nutrition info for you. If you're not sure how many calories something has, look it up online. And if you're not sure of the amount you ate, take your best guess.

You'll never be perfect with counting calories so don't try to be. When you're unsure of something, take your best guess and move on. Soon enough you'll get a good feel for how you need to eat in order to lose weight or build muscle. You can use the eyeball test to get a good estimate quickly once this happens. Until you reach that point, make sure that you diligently track your calories for the best results possible.

What Foods Should I Eat?

It's no surprise that you need to eat clean, high-quality calories in order to see the best results you can. Getting your calories in by eating ice cream and potato chips isn't going to have the same effect on your body like fruits and vegetables will.

If you want more specifics on how you should be eating and what to eat, be sure to check out my other books. I have written about many of the best nutritional strategies in existence today, so find what works best for you and do it. I believe that flexible dieting and intermittent fasting are the best nutritional approaches out there, and they're a great place to start if you're not sure where to begin.

One final tip—do not obsess over trying to eat healthy 100% of the time. This is unrealistic for most people. Imagine if you go to a birthday party or you have a catered lunch at your job. What are you going to do? Look like a health nut and say, "No thanks, I'm good with my chicken breast and brown rice." No.

What you should do instead is commit to eating healthy 85% of the time. This is plenty good enough for you to still be able to get great results. It'll also take a lot of pressure off of you to be perfect all of the time. And best of all, it'll give you leeway to be able to eat with your friends and family during social events like parties and weddings!

Chapter 9: Do You Need to Do Cardio With Your Strength Training Routine?

The short answer to this is that you can if you want to, but you certainly don't have to. It depends on what your goals are. If you want to burn fat, doing the right type of cardio can help you out. If you're trying to build muscle, cardio might interfere more than it helps depending on how you do it.

Regardless of if you decide to do cardio or not, always (and I mean always) do it on a rest day or after you complete your strength-training workout. By doing the cardio first, you'll fatigue yourself and you won't be able to lift as much as you could if you were fresh.

Is Cardio Even Necessary to Burn Fat?

No matter what anyone else tells you, you don't have to do cardio to burn fat. I can completely understand why many people think that they must do hours upon hours of cardio if they want to shred a few pounds.

You hear all of the time about how fitness models and bodybuilders use cardio as a way to get absolutely shredded, so it's easy to believe that it's necessary. However, cardio is not required at all to lose weight and get down to a low level of body fat.

What is required to lose weight and shred fat is a caloric deficit as I have already mentioned earlier. It doesn't matter if you use exercise (i.e. cardio in this case) and/or diet to get into a caloric deficit. Both will get the job done.

It's much easier to control your total number of calories through your diet as opposed to exercising more. Think about it for a second.

What's easier—eating a slice of pizza and then doing 30 minutes of cardio to burn it off, or not eating the slice of pizza in the first place? It's obvious; you shouldn't eat the pizza in the first place.

Sure, you could try to burn off the extra calories every now and then, but it won't last for long. You're just fighting an uphill battle because 30 minutes of your time isn't worth whatever it is that you want to eat so badly.

That's why you hear people say that you can't out-exercise a bad diet. It is true, so focus more on your diet and the number of calories that you're eating rather than doing more cardio.

Also, don't fret if you think this means that you'll have to give up your favorite foods to lose weight. It doesn't. You'll still get to enjoy your favorite foods *without* having to worry about weight gain or doing some extra cardio to make up for it.

A New Way to Think About Cardio

From now on, think about cardio as a tool that can help you burn some extra calories instead of thinking of it as a requirement to lose weight. Cardio is one way to help get you into a caloric deficit, and you can use it when you feel that it's needed to get the job done.

Just like how a single tool usually won't be enough to get the job done, cardio alone usually won't be enough to get you into a caloric deficit. You still need to focus on your nutrition plan.

With this type of mindset, you'll only have to do cardio when you feel that it's necessary. It's important to remember that cardio isn't required in order for you to start seeing jaw-dropping results.

I believe that honing in on nutrition is the right way to go when trying to lose weight. This is because diet is the easiest and fastest way to control the total number of calories you're eating.

However, once you have your diet in check, if you feel like adding in some extra exercise then do so. Cardio can be a good way to speed up the fat loss process, or give you more leeway in your diet.

The Best Cardio Workout

With so many cardio workouts in existence today, which one is the best? Is it a slow steady state cardio?

How about sprinting? Or maybe any type of cardio done on an empty stomach is the best?

The kind of cardio that you do isn't as important as simply doing it. So I would first and foremost recommend doing any type of cardio you enjoy, whether that's walking, sprinting, jogging, or a mix of all three. However, I will say the cardio workout I'll be providing you with here is the best way to go.

It's a combination of high intensity interval training (HIIT) and slow steady state cardio. Research has shown higher intensity cardio results in more fat loss over time than lower intensity cardio (11) (12).

HIIT really is efficient—you're burning more calories in less time. HIIT is even better when combined with slow steady state cardio.

The reason why is because the HIIT will release free fatty acids into the bloodstream, and then the slow steady state cardio will burn off those free fatty acids.

Most people will do HIIT but won't follow it up with slow steady state cardio. This is really a shame because all of those free fatty acids released into the bloodstream will just get reabsorbed.

Here's how to do a combo cardio workout:

Note: This cardio workout can be done on any type of cardio machine (treadmill, elliptical, etc.), outside, on a track, or wherever else you want. The workout will be the same.

Combo Cardio Workout

10-15 minutes of HIIT on treadmill (or cardio machine of choice)

-Sprint for 30 seconds

-Walk for 1 minute (alternate between sprinting and walking for the full 10-15 min)

Immediately followed by: 10-15 minutes of steady state cardio

-Walk on treadmill at 3.5 mph

Now the cool thing about HIIT is that you can adjust it to your current fitness level. For example if you can't sprint for 30 seconds, do a fast jog for 20 seconds (7.5 mph on a treadmill as an example) and then walk for 1 minute and 10 seconds.

You could even do 45 seconds of sprinting and 45 seconds of walking if you're in better shape. You can customize it to your needs, but you have the do the HIIT first, and then follow it up with the slow steady state cardio.

I recommend that you do this 20-30 minute workout 2-3 times per week. I wouldn't advise that you do it anymore than this because that's too much, and it's unnecessary at that point.

Final Thoughts on Cardio

You might not feel like doing HIIT sometimes. What do you do then? Luckily you don't have to skip cardio altogether—there's an easier way and it's called walking. I recommend walking as much as you possibly can.

Walking is great because it can help to reduce stress (13) and speed up recovery from a hard workout. Walking also helps with lymphatic system recovery, and there's research showing how walking more (or just moving more in general for that matter) can reduce your risk for developing heart disease (14).

Best of all, walking is an easy way to burn more calories. I used to think that walking was only for people who weren't in that good of shape, but boy was I wrong about that!

Walking should be done by everyone, fit or unfit. The simple fact is that walking provides benefits that the higher intensity cardio just can't.

I recommend going for walks around town or at the local park. Go outside and get some fresh air.

Walking for 30 minutes 3 days a week would be enough to start providing you with some amazing benefits. You can still do the combination cardio workout twice per week in addition to the walking if you want to, or do walking only.

Chapter 10: Frequently Asked Questions

What if I'm not gaining weight eating the amount of calories you recommend?

In order to start gaining weight and build muscle I advise the following:

Bodyweight x 13 + 250 = total daily calories.

Let's say a couple of weeks have gone by, and you haven't been gaining any weight. What should you do? You'll want to continue to add in an additional 100 calories every week until you start gaining weight. Let's use an example with a 110-pound individual:

Body weight = 110 pounds
110 x 13 = 1,430
1,430 + 250 = 1,680

After 1 week of no weight gain:
1,680 + 100 = 1,780

This means the individual will now eat 1,780 calories, and if she doesn't gain any weight, she'll bump it up again as follows for the next week:

After 2 weeks of no weight gain:
1,780 + 100 = 1,880

After 3 week of no weight gain:

1,880 + 100 = 1,980

You would continue doing this until you reach the sweet spot of gaining roughly half a pound per week.

What if I'm not losing weight eating 13 calories per pound of bodyweight?

If you've been struggling to lose weight eating 13 calories per pound of bodyweight, I recommend using a different method to set your calories. Before I get into that though, you must first make sure you were actually eating 13 calories per pound of body weight minus 500 calories to lose 1 pound per week. It's easy to overestimate the amount of calories you're eating, and this could be the reason why you're not seeing results.

Once you've made sure you've accurately been tracking your calories, you can take your goal bodyweight, multiply it by 11, and then eat that many calories (don't subtract anything from the final calculated number).

Yes, I understand that your goal bodyweight will be a random number that you think you'll look good at, so take your best guess. Start on the higher side and work your way down from there if you still aren't losing weight.

Here's an example for a 170-pound female.

Current Weight 170

Goal Body weight 150

200 x 11 = 1,650 daily calories

Let's say that once this person reaches her goal of 150 pounds she's still not satisfied with how she looks. From there, she can simply set a new goal bodyweight (i.e. 140 pounds for example) and go from there.

What if I hit a plateau and I stop losing weight at my regular pace?

Let's say you've been losing weight just fine, but then all of the sudden you hit a wall and stop losing weight. In this case, take your new current body weight (which should be a lower number from when you first started) and multiply that by 13.

Take that number and subtract 250 from it. This will be your new daily caloric intake for you to lose weight.

This will have you losing weight at a rate of approximately 0.5-pound per week. You may have previously been losing weight at a rate of 1-pound per week, but now you'll lose at a rate of 0.5-pound per week.

This is because I don't want you to drastically reduce your calories all of a sudden; if you've hit a plateau, you're likely very close to hitting your goal weight anyway.

How many meals should I eat per day?

You can eat as many meals as you like throughout the day. Meal frequency doesn't matter for weight loss (15), but the total amount of calories you eat does. So eat however many is easiest for you and your schedule.

I prefer to eat 3 meals a day, and that works great for most other people too. However, feel free to eat 6 times per day or even as little as once per day. As long as you're hitting your macros, you'll be fine.

What do I do once I reach my goal bodyweight?

Contrary to what you might be thinking, things aren't going to be that much different from what you've been doing to lose weight. You still need to follow your nutrition plan and continue eating in the same manner that you previously were. This means that you should still keep the same eating schedule and keep eating similar meals to the ones that you were eating to lose weight.

However, there's one difference between maintenance and creating a caloric deficit to lose weight. The difference is that you get to consume more calories! How many calories? Well, this is pretty easy to figure out as a matter of fact.

Step #1: Determine at what rate you were losing weight (i.e. 1 pound per week)

Step #2: Translate pounds lost per week into calories
0.5-pound lost per week = 250 calories
1 pound lost per week = 500 calories
1.5 pounds lost per week = 750 calories
2 pounds lost per week = 1,000 calories, etc.

Step #3: Add in those additional calories to what you were previously eating to maintain your new weight.

For example, let's say someone was losing weight at a rate of 1 pound per week by eating 1,850 calories per day. Once she hits her goal weight, she needs to eat 2,350 calories (1,850+500) per day to maintain her new weight.

Can you go over how much weight I should be lifting during the workouts again?

Lift as much weight as you possibly can for the given rep range. Initially, you won't know how much weight to use, so you'll have to take your best guess. For example, let's say you're doing bench press for 8 reps. You think you can lift around 150 pounds for that many reps, but on your first set, you easily complete 10 reps.

This means the weight is too light and you need to increase it for the next set. On the next set, you lift 165 pounds and struggle to complete the 8th rep. This is what you want to happen, and it means you've found a good weight to use. Once you can complete all 3 sets for 8 reps with 165 pounds, move up to 170 the next time you bench press. If you can't complete 8 reps for all 3 sets, stick with 165 until you can. Here's an example:

Workout 1: Bench Press with 165 pounds
Set 1: 8 reps
Set 2: 8 reps
Set 3: 7 reps

Because you only completed 7 reps on the last set, stick with 165 for the next workout.

Workout 2: Bench Press with 165 pounds
Set 1: 8 reps
Set 2: 8 reps
Set 3: 8 reps

Because you completed all 3 sets for 8 reps, move up to 170 on your next workout with bench press.

Note: It's better to use a weight that's too heavy and miss a rep or two than it is to use a weight that's too light and leave some reps in the tank. For example, it's better to do 170 pounds and only complete 6 reps out of 8 as opposed to using 155 pounds and stopping at 8 reps even though you could've easily done more reps.

How Fast Should I Lose Weight?

The more weight you have to lose, the faster the rate at which you can lose the weight. For example, if you have 50+

pounds to lose, you can lose weight at a rate of 2 pounds or more per week. If you only have 5 pounds to lose, then lose weight at a rate of 0.5 pound per week.

For most people, losing 1 pound per week is the sweet spot. You'll be creating an average caloric deficit of 500 calories daily. At this pace, you'll be losing weight fairly quickly, and you won't be miserable all of the time from a complete lack of calories.

How much water should I drink on a daily basis?

Your body is made up of about 60% water so it's important to consume water for several reasons. Drinking water regularly:

- Helps keep your joints and ligaments fluid, which can help prevent injury
- Helps control your caloric intake
- Flushes out toxins
- Improves skin quality
- Improves kidney function
- Improves your focus

Many people recommend that you should drink 1 gallon of water per day. This is a blanket answer that doesn't meet individual needs. This recommendation would have a 100-pound woman drinking the same amount of water as a 200-pound man. Absurd!

Other health experts advise drinking eight 8-ounce glasses (64 ounces total) of water a day. But again 64 ounces isn't going to be enough for most people. What should you do then? I don't keep track of my water intake—I go by how I feel and the color of my urine.

Your body's own thirst mechanism will be accurate in telling you if you need more water. If you feel thirsty, go drink some water. If not, then you're probably ok. You can also use the color of your urine to judge how hydrated you are. If your urine is yellow, then you should drink more water. If it's clear then you should be good to go. This keeps things simple and it's one less thing you have to keep track of.

Are there any supplements that you recommend I take?

Most supplements are a complete waste of money. There's not a single supplement that's required in order for you to build muscle or burn fat. In fact, I advise for the first 6 weeks of your training program that you don't take *any* supplements at all.

This is because I want you to see for yourself that it really is possible for you to get results without supplements. Your hard work and dedication matter way more than any pill or powder.

With that being said, there are a few supplements I recommend if you have the budget for them:

#1: Protein Powder:

You can't have a recommended list of supplements without protein powder on the list right? Just kidding. But this has to be one of the most overhyped supplements of all time.

I think that the media does a really good job of making us believe that we must take protein powder to build muscle or take it to prevent muscle loss. I do think that protein powder can provide some benefits if *you need it.*

If you struggle to consistently hit your macros with protein then I would consider investing in a protein powder. Protein is necessary to help build and prevent the breakdown of muscle.

Therefore, ensuring that your muscle is spared is a good thing. However, don't go out of your way and eat more calories just for the sake of consuming more protein.

#2: Fish/Krill Oil

These oils are great sources of Omega-3 fatty acids. This is a good thing because most people consume too many Omega-6 fatty acids with foods like vegetable and canola oil.

Ideally, you want to be consuming a 1 to 1 ratio of Omega-3's to Omega-6's. Fish and krill oil can help you narrow the gap between the two types of fatty acids that you're consuming.

The main benefit from consuming these oils is that they act as an anti-inflammatory in your body. When you consume Omega-6's on the other hand, they act as an inflammatory.

That's why it's important to strike a balance with both of the fatty acids. The anti-inflammatory benefit is great because it can reduce your risk of developing heart disease or high blood pressure.

Finally, reducing inflammation can aid in muscle recovery. If you're going to invest in fish or krill oil, make sure that it's a very high-grade supplement.

The way that some of the lower quality oils are processed inhibits the absorption of them, which would make them completely useless. As for investing in fish or krill oil, taking either one is fine really.

Krill oil does contain the antioxidant astaxanthin (16), which helps with joint health, boosts cognitive function and helps promote a healthy cholesterol balance, while fish oil does not. However, I have noticed that krill oil can be harder to find, and it's typically more expensive, so don't sweat not buying it.

#3: Digestive Enzymes

This is my favorite supplement of all time, and it's probably one of the most underrated supplements as well. If your body can't absorb the vitamins and nutrients that you're consuming, then what's the point?

The sad fact of the matter is that when our foods get cooked, many of the enzymes get destroyed. Digestive enzymes will not only help to replenish those enzymes missed from cooked foods, but it will also help your body to better break down and utilize the nutrients that you're eating.

Also, if you ever suffer regularly from bloating, heartburn, or have bad skin, give digestive enzymes a try and see if you notice a difference. Of course, it's important to note that these enzymes need to be high quality if you want them to be of any use.

Simply going to the local grocery store and purchasing a $10 bottle of enzymes isn't going to cut it. You must buy a high-quality enzyme if you want to get any use out of it.

How Do I Motivate Myself to Go to the Gym?

Finding the motivation to go to the gym or eat right can be hard. No matter who you are, there will be times when you don't feel like working out. Having that feeling is ok, but you can't let it control you. There will be times when you'll have to do it anyway even when you don't feel like it.

That's what will ultimately separate a long-term successful fitness journey from failing at it. I do have some tips to help you out along the way however:

Tip #1: Focus on Gradual Improvements

Many people make fitness an all-or-nothing game. They tell themselves that they'll workout 5 days a week and eat clean 100% of the time for the rest of their lives. Let's say you workout only 4 days one week. Are you a failure?

Of course not. You still worked out 4 days, but in your mind you are because you failed to reach 5 workouts. You make it hard to celebrate any small successes that you do have because the standards are too high.

Instead, focus on making smaller, more gradual improvements, and celebrate any successes you have along the way. For example, start off with a goal to only workout 2 days per week if it's been years since you've last worked out. Once you achieve that goal, you'll feel good about yourself, and you can move up to working out 3 days per week and so on.

Tip #2: Action Leads Motivation

People think they have to get the inspiration or motivation from somewhere in order to take the action necessary to workout. The reverse of that is actually true. You need to start by taking an action no matter how small. And once you get started, you'll likely want to continue on with what you're doing.

When I think about everything I have to do to workout such as put my gym clothes on, drive to the gym, workout with a bunch of grueling exercises, drive back and shower, I start to make up silly excuses as to why I should skip this time. Instead, I'll tell myself to do just one exercise when I get to the gym and not pressure myself to do anything more. After I finish that first exercise, it's always easier for me to finish the rest of the workout.

You just have to get started. Try this out for any healthy habit you want to start. For example, if you want to start flossing your teeth, tell yourself you'll only floss one tooth and don't pressure yourself to do anything more than that!

Tip #3: Put Your Own Money on the Line

Money is a very powerful motivator, and you can use your own money to motivate yourself to start working out more. Here's what you're going to do—give someone a good amount of money. Not $20, but something that would actually hurt you—$100, $200, $500, or whatever you can't afford to lose.

Then tell your friend that if you don't go to the gym 3 days this week, for example, they get to keep the money. When you give up the money in the first place, you'll fight to get it back. This is much different than telling yourself you'll give the money to someone after you miss your workouts.

It's too easy to make an excuse and not give away the money. Give the money up in the first place and make sure your friend actually holds you accountable to it. This is by far the best way to get motivation to workout. There's a real cost involved if you don't comply. You'll either get ripped or go broke trying.

Conclusion

Thank you so much for reading this book all the way to the end! All that's left to do now is execute! You could have all of the knowledge in the world about the latest and greatest training techniques, but it won't do you any good unless you take action! You can do it and achieve great things if you put your mind to it. Good luck!

Finally be sure to download the video guide where I personally demonstrate how to perform all of the exercises by visiting the link directly below:

http://rohmerfitness.com/womenvideoguide

And if you have any other questions please be sure to email me at thomas@rohmerfitness.com. I'd be more than happy to answer any fitness questions you have!

Sources

(1) https://en.wikipedia.org/wiki/Testosterone

(2) https://www.muscleforlife.com/turn-fat-into-muscle/

(3) https://www.ncbi.nlm.nih.gov/pubmed/10198297

(4) https://www.ncbi.nlm.nih.gov/pubmed/18090659

(5) https://www.ncbi.nlm.nih.gov/pubmed/20020365

(6) https://www.ncbi.nlm.nih.gov/pubmed/25853914

(7)
http://www.sciencedirect.com/science/article/pii/07495978
87900458

(8) https://en.wikipedia.org/wiki/Egocentric_predicament

(9) https://www.ncbi.nlm.nih.gov/pubmed/25268291

(10) https://www.ncbi.nlm.nih.gov/pubmed/22825659

(11) http://www.ncbi.nlm.nih.gov/pubmed/20473222

(12) http://www.ncbi.nlm.nih.gov/pubmed/18197184

(13) http://www.ncbi.nlm.nih.gov/pubmed/18787373

(14)
http://www.health.harvard.edu/newsletter_article/Walking-Your-steps-to-health

(15) https://www.ncbi.nlm.nih.gov/pubmed/26024494

(16) https://en.wikipedia.org/wiki/Astaxanthin